The scope of avascular necrosis in the vertebral spine

C. Panow MD

Printed by CreateSpace

"An insolent reply from a polite person is a bad sign".

Hippocrates (460-370BC)

Disclaimer

The author and publisher decline responsibility about any deleterious effect resulting from wrong understanding or misinterpretation of present text.

This publication is meant for information purposes only.

Key words

Avascular necrosis, bone necrosis, hypovitaminosis, osteochondrosis, Kümmel's disease, Schmorl's node, Vitamin D, bone density, bone vascularity.

Avascular necrosis (AVN) of the vertebral spine has many facets.

Multiplicity of factors

The first interesting fact, to be aware of, is that AVN can be due to a large variety of underlying diseases.

Etiologies as different as vascular compromise, inflammation, hormonal disturbances, vitamin deficiencies and congenital disease make up the scope of AVN of bone.

Sickle cell disease, vasculitis, anti-phospholipid syndrome, systemic lupus erythematosus, Gaucher's disease, muco-poly-saccharidoses, Ehlers-Danlos disease, scurvy, rickets, caisson disease, fat embolism, hyper-lipo-proteinemias, some medication as for instance anti-retroviral therapy, steroidal and non-steroidal anti-

inflammatory drugs, pregnancy, pancreatitis, pancreatic carcinoma, alcoholism, Cushing's disease, organ transplantation, radiotherapy, trauma, electrical shock, myelogenous leukemia, Langerhans'cell histiocytosis and tumor have all been reported as possible causes.
2,4,5,7,10,13,16,18,19,20,21,23

Several synonyms have been used in the past to coin this phenomenon.

Terminology

Avascular necrosis is nowadays the most widely accepted term.

Aseptic necrosis is still used in some texts.

This term was initially meant to differentiate the entity from bone necrosis induced by osteomyelitis.

8

Specific context of osteomyelitis

Necrotic bone parts and fragments in an infectious context are called involucrum and sequestrum, which have been the first manifestations of bone necrosis to be described with radiography. [14]

This has been also historically the first situation in which necrosis in the skeleton has been observed, correctly interpreted and reported precisely in medical literature as such in 18th century already.

Interpretation of X-Rays

Initially radiologists recognized the higher density of necrotic fragments on radiographs, but failed to realize for about 80 years, until tomodensitometry became available, that it is not necrotic bone which is hyper-dense, but surrounding bone which becomes osteopenic as a result of secondary hyperemia and resorption.

Necrotic bone is actually the only part which is not involved in the reparative process, being cut away from vascular supply. Thus the term avascular necrosis.

In the vertebral spine AVN manifests itself in several ways.

Reports by radiologists

Some features are known since a long time:

The first reports occurred within a few years after Röntgen's discovery of X-rays.[14]

Other aspects are depicted only since clinical application of modern imaging techniques, especially since MRI exists. [2,6,9,11,13,20,21,23]

Our knowledge will certainly progress with more extensive use of this modality.

Those lessons, which we inherit from past history and progression of present knowledge, teach us that we can only speculate, how much remains still to be discovered and described about AVN and its imaging characteristics.

Until now several *imaging features* in the vertebral spine have been well documented.

Vertebral periphery

Scheuermann's disease

The first of them, to be reported in world literature, concerns manifestations of disease at the periphery of vertebral bodies.

This aspect should be understood as a reparative process, observed some time after the responsible event, rather than being an acute finding (Drawings 2-6).

One example of this phenomenon are *Schmorl's nodes*.

They can affect any location of the vertebral plate, and are easily distinguished in this respect from notochord rests which are limited to the posterior third of the vertebra, in a central location.

Off-center depressions or such involving anterior

two thirds of vertebral plateaus are thus diagnostic of Schmorl's nodes.

Schmorl's nodes have been initially reported in *Scheuermann's disease*, but can also be seen with a similar shape in other pathological settings, especially such associated with *osteoporosis, or trauma.* [15]

The clinical context and associated findings allow distinction between these different entities in daily practice.

Osteoporosis

Osteoporosis is classically associated with a «fish vertebra» appearance of vertebral bodies, probably another manifestation of bone necrosis, the result of regular give-away of vertebral plateaus to body weight.

Sometimes MRI shows pathological enhancement adjacent to an indented vertebral plate, an observation which supports the hypothesis of AVN as intermediate phenomenon leading to biconcave configuration.

Whether result of osteonecrosis or fracture of trabecular scaffold, «fish vertebra» deformation of vertebral plates in osteoporosis seems to be sub-acute or chronic, rather than a result of an acute event, as result of adaptation to mechanical stress.

It appears usually within 10-14 days after minor trauma.

Irregularities of vertebral plates

Vertebral size

On the other hand Scheuermann's disease shows

in most cases other reparative findings such as irregularities of vertebral plateaus and deformity of affected vertebrae. (Fig 3-6)

In some cases of Scheuermann's disease cortical outlines of affected vertebral bodies have outgrown antero-posterior or transverse diameters of their neighbor vertebrae.

This feature signs chronology and chronicity of responsible mechanism, which must have taken place during adolescence, i.e. towards end of skeletal growing.

Another feature of Scheuermann's disease is cuneiform deformation of vertebral bodies.

Recent advances in vitamin deficiencies research indicates that Scheuermann's disease is probably end-result of rickets.

In this respect osteoporosis is ultimate image of osteomalacia (Chronic vitamin D deficiency, rickets being sub-acute or acute deficit in infancy and childhood of this vitamin).

Congenital diseases

Similar findings to those of Scheuermann's disease have been observed in other, especially congenital diseases:

-    For instance, *progressive pseudo-rheumatoid arthritis of childhood* and some bone dysplasias can present with similar features.

-    In this last group *spondyloepiphyseal dysplasia tarda (SEDT)* has been reported with characteristics in the vertebral spine almost indistinguishable from those of Scheuermann's disease.

The responsible process in SEDT though is in most

cases more severe, accompanied by deficient trunk growth, ending in small stature. [10]

Relation to Perthes disease

Hip lesions in SEDT are similar to those of Perthes' disease, a fact that further militates for a role of AVN in this type of dysplasia.

For many reasons radiography of the lumbar spine should include the hip joint, one of these being that some rare patients presenting with signs of "Scheuermann's disease" in the vertebral spine turn out to have «flattening» of the femoral heads, and thus represent probably a form of SEDT.

Rather than being one homogeneous entity, this type of dysplasia could represent, like other similar illnesses, several congenital defects, not identified individually as such by modern medicine as yet.

It can be speculated that probably only one defect or some of the cases of SEDT resemble truly Scheuermann's disease.

Anterior displacement of nucleus pulposus, accompanied by indentation of anterior third of vertebral plateaus has been described in SEDT as having imaging similarities with Schmorl's nodes of Scheuermann's disease.

Vertebral plates are grossly irregular in SEDT, and vertebral outlines deformed, with large antero-posterior diameters of vertebral bodies.

On the other hand, at the end of the spectrum, a common manifestation of SEDT is platyspondyly, which is very similar to Calvé's osteochondrosis, and thus implies a common physiopathological pathway.

Osteochondroses and rickets

Within similar logic, most osteochondroses are probably due to rickets.

In cases where etiology of Schmorl's nodes remains undetermined despite thorough analysis of associated findings, MRI can help distinguish Scheuermann's disease from osteoporosis.

In the latter indistinct margins and peripheral contrast enhancement of Schmorl's nodes are signs of recently evolving lesions.

In first mentioned entity such an observation should be expected only during maximal growth of adolescence.

On the other hand bone sclerosis and smooth outlines are features of a longer standing, old process.

Thus AVN plays a role in vertebral body deformation observed in many different settings.

The case of osteoporosis

Osteoporosis manifests itself on radiography as accentuation and coarsening of vertical trabecular scaffold comparatively to the rest of cancellous bone and also as a relative accentuation of vertebral plateaus in comparison to the medullary space. [16]

In fact, this feature means relative paucity of trabecular irregular medullary bone, rather than increase in number or thickness of vertical pillars and perpendicular cortical plates.

If we observe such signs of osteoporosis in an elderly patient, in the context of acute vertebral pain, especially after a minor trauma, we can prompt further investigation.

Control after a few weeks, even if the first radiograph didn't disclose any traumatic abnormality, has frequently showed cuneiform vertebral body deformation.

Kümmel's disease

This phenomenon is due to *Kümmel's disease*, another manifestation of AVN in the vertebral spine.

MRI can disclose a focus of bone necrosis before any abnormalities are visible on conventional radiographs.

Some invasive techniques trying to prevent or reverse spinal height loss, have been described, but end with modest results.

Thus flattening of vertebral bodies, when established, should be considered for the moment as definitive, out of the spectrum of reasonable modern therapy.

Instruction by a trained orthopedic surgeon should be sought, in order to avoid dealing with a true compression fracture, which ends-up unstable.

In Kümmel's disease posterior vertebral elements are rarely, if ever, involved in shrinking process, and thus, what is called frequently in medical facilities "compression fracture" of the elderly, is uncommonly completely unstable.

AVN as common disease

AVN considered to be post-traumatic in the context of osteoporosis in elderly patients is a common entity, and has been described long ago by H. Kümmel. [7]

His description almost coincided with discovery of X-rays by W. Röntgen.

Though well defined, Kümmel's disease seems frequently forgotten or ignored in modern imaging, and sometimes completely misunderstood and wrongly interpreted as a fracture.

Vertebral body height loss in Kümmel's disease occurs typically delayed relative to the initiating minor traumatic event, in contradistinction to vertebral body fracture where deformation is immediately visible.

This phenomenon represents also the explanation for overall diminishing body height in elderly people and can't be considered a rare syndrome.

Restrictive use of modern radiological modalities, and especially MR, has kept us from realizing all imaging features of Kümmel's disease in our «modern» environment.

The case of vertebra plana

Vertebra plana had originally been described by *J. Calvé* as osteochondrosis of the primary ossification center of the vertebral body, comparable to that of the femoral head observed in Perthes disease. [4]

Different eponyms shouldn't mask understanding of common physiopathological pathways.

It is important to realize that Kümmel, Calvé and Perthes have described the same phenomenon and thus coined it with a different terminology whether it manifests itself in the vertebral spine or in the femoral head, in adulthood or childhood.

One of the main differential diagnoses of vertebra plana is *Langerhans' cell histiocytosis* of bone, previously known as eosinophilic granuloma in its solitary form and as Hand-Schüller-Christian's disease in its multilocular variant.

The role of AVN in this setting seems obvious, though being the subject of few reports with modern imaging modalities.

Central gas inclusions in the vertebral bodies, visible on conventional radiographs and T2-hyperintensities in the same location depicted with MRI, have been described between the first specific imaging signs of AVN in the spine.

These publications concerned though cases where

important vertebral body height loss had already occurred, almost similar to a vertebra plana.

On the other hand, there is a paucity of radiological reports on early signs of AVN in the spine.

The case of sickle cell anemia

Sickle cell anemia (SCA), homozygous form for S-hemoglobin, causes the red blood cells to assume an elongated configuration under conditions of reduced oxygen pressure in blood.

This sickle cell configuration results in mechanical capillary stasis rather than thrombosis, and leads to hypoxic damage in tissues.

Features of consecutive bone changes look like Legg-Calvé-Perthes' disease, so it is easy to assume similar physiopathology.

Vertebrae in SCA deform themselves, resembling compression fractures.

Typical characteristics in this disease are cuneiform deformation and vertebral body height loss, even leading to vertebra plana.

Biconcave or «fish vertebra» deformation observed also in SCA is assumed to be rather due to bone marrow proliferation with secondary rarefication and bone loss.

Previous remarks about osteoporosis and biconcave deformation apply also to this disease.

Such way of thinking would imply that excessive bone marrow proliferation could be another promoting factor of AVN.

What about other hemoglobinopathies accompanied frequently by «fish vertebra» deformation of the vertebral bodies?

Other Hemopathies

For instance multiple myeloma typically manifests this way.

Unfortunately reports in medical literature about this topic are rather scarce, owing to a certain reluctance of primary care physicians to use modern imaging techniques in illnesses which they consider «well known».

On the other hand this behavior is explained by the very much stressed modern concept of «cost efficient medicine».

Unfortunately, not infrequently, moderate costs

imply moderate efficiency of medical undertaking.

AVN and Infection

AVN lesions, as any necrotic tissue, demonstrate reduced defense towards microorganisms.

The result is relative frequency of osteomyelitis, with unusual features in the vertebral spine in this context.

In contradistinction to usual spondylodiscitis, which initially affects the intervertebral disc and only secondarily involves adjacent vertebral plates, and then bodies, salmonella infection of the vertebral spine in sickle cell disease seldom affects the intervertebral disc.

Thus it seems obvious that this kind of infection doesn't originate in the intervertebral disc, but is primarily a bone process: - Result of AVN!

Chronic salmonella infection has a prevalence of up to 50% in SCA, probably owing to increased Hemoglobin turnover.

As in other hemoglobinopathies bilirubin gallstones and sludge in the gallbladder are formed, which serve as support to a chronic carrying state of bacterias and especially salmonellas.[12]

Prevalence depends also on local geographic factors, because of differences in strain distribution, some salmonella types being much more virulent than others.

Chronic salmonella infection is rare or even unknown in some countries, owing probably to different soil characteristics.

It is rare in Western Europe, most cases in

Geneva, where I am working, coming from the Middle East.

AVN and Spleen

Other pathogens are also responsible for osteomyelitis in sickle cell disease, host defenses being reduced for several reasons and especially because of functional asplenia:

- Streptococcus pneumoniae and Klebsiella pneumoniae, as well as Staphylococcus aureus are thus also commonly encountered.

Bacterias encapsulated with polysaccharide coating are responsible for severe, highly lethal septicemic infections in patients without a functional spleen.

Thus, such individuals should be treated

aggressively with antibiotics if pneumococcal pneumonia or some other infection implying this kind of germs is considered on clinical grounds.

Here again, it is probably ischemic bouts owing to repeated spleen infarction which end-up in functional asplenia.

Vascular rheological factors as well as extra-medullary hematopoiesis and increased breakdown of red blood cells play a role in repeated spleen infarction and subsequent fibrosis.

While flare up of infections and acute infarction induce moderate splenomegaly, extramedullary hematopoiesis can promote important spleen growth to over 1 liter (33oz volume), the end-result of a long lasting sickle cell disease being still frequently a small scarred spleen.

Unusual aspect of AVN should raise suspicion

Extensive use of imaging techniques and especially MRI, PET and SPECT would make radiologists more familiar with typical features of bone AVN.

Unusual imaging findings which seem out of the scope of AVN, especially in the setting of sickle cell disease, or in patients otherwise at risk for septic complications, should make consider secondary spondylitis and prompt emergently further investigation and treatment in this setting.

Soft tissue enhancement doesn't belong to AVN of bone and thus any paravertebral modification should be considered with suspicion.

Sub-periosteal or epidural fluid collection, or thickening and enhancement of soft tissue can mean abscess formation or evolving phlegmone, and are carriers of separate prognostic gravity.

Gadolinium-enhanced MRI, PET, SPECT as well as Gallium- and Technetium-Scintigraphy have all an important role to play in this regard.

Importance of MRI

MRI remains probably most important because of wide availability of technique in industrialized countries, good feasibility, as well as high diagnostic yield with appropriate protocols.

Un-adapted sequences however, and especially non-Gadolinium-enhanced MRI scans, on the other hand, can be misleading, failing to demonstrate infection at hand.

Bone within bone

Pediatric radiologists sometimes observe an image called «bone within bone», or in the vertebral spine «*vertebra-in-vertebra*», which is interpreted as end-result of various noxious stimuli.

Patients sometimes recall an episode of serious illness which has taken place during infancy or childhood.

Size of the inner vertebral shape allows a precise chronological location of the responsible event.

This process leaves a shadow of vertebral outlines inside the further growing vertebral body.

Such a phenomenon could find its explanation in necrotic bone, which doesn't contain viable cells any more, and thus was unable to resorb completely its solid and tough cortical boundaries, while periosteal bone deposition and vertebral growth progressed further.

We can only speculate whether all illnesses

reported in relation with a «vertebra-in-vertebra» appearance, and which are varied, result from AVN;

- Such a fact would blow-up considerably the etiological span of bone necrosis, including thus sepsis, shock and malnutrition between a vast number of other «serious illnesses» and causes in its scope.

Neuropathic disease

Neuropathic disease (ND) is another situation, where bone necrosis could play a role, though not initially.

This entity presents with very peculiar articular changes accompanied by bone fragmentation, the process being characterized by absent or minor reparative features.

Such ND can be observed in the spine, mainly in

the context of syringo-myelia, neuro-syphilis, but most frequently due to vitamin B12-deficit in elderly people, in conjunction with degeneration of posterior tracts of myelon.

ND of other etiologies manifests in the extremities, most frequently due to diabetes mellitus and vitamin B12-deficit, the first being accompanied by only faint changes in axial skeleton.

Central pathological importance in ND is attributed to the joint itself, which seems to be first structure affected, articular space narrowing and eburnation preceding usually bone fragmentation.

Sinusoidal type of AVN

Gaucher's disease, mucopolysaccharidoses, Langerhans' cell histiocytosis X and metastases could induce AVN probably by impeding venous return due to diffuse bone marrow infiltration.

Restriction of the usually abundant sinusoidal bed ensues, which can increase intra-osseous hydrostatic pressure and reduce collateral flow reserves.

Batson's venous plexus could probably explain some cases of venous retrograde embolization with pathological cells.

Pancreas

Hydrolytic enzymes shedding in the blood flow and especially lipases secreted in pancreatic disease are probably responsible for bone necrosis in this setting:

-    AVN has been observed in pancreatitis and some pancreatic tumors as well.

Direct toxic effect of enzymatic tissue damage plays probably initially a decisive role.

Secondary hyperlipidemia due to lipolysis, with consecutive lipid embolization has been advanced as one hypothesis of responsible mechanism.

Even as we start realizing the frequency of AVN, its precise **physiopathology** still remains obscure in many situations, and we can only suppose that demand of oxygen and nutriments outweighs supply at the moment of acute event.

Embolism

In many situations evidence prevails as to an embolic etiology, this being the case not only for vasculitis and collagen vascular diseases, but also for a series of situations where fat embolism either due to hyper-lipo-proteinemia, i.e. in anti-retroviral therapy, or induced fat catabolism, as in corticosteroid therapy and alcoholism is postulated.

Further any infiltrative process of the medullary space, either by phagocytic cells as in various storage diseases, or by hematopoietic, inflammatory or even neoplastic cells, or simply by increased amount of yellow, that is fat marrow, diminishes the size of the usually extensive network of sinusoids, impedes collateral blood flow and could favor osteonecrosis.

Corticosteroids

Thus corticosteroid therapy, for instance, can favor AVN through several mechanisms:

- Fat involution;
- Lipid embolism;
- Osteoporosis;
- Catabolic effect...

Hydrostatic pressure within cancellous bone seems to depend on many factors and its increase can of course also tighten blood flow reserves.

Inflammatory response due to any damage of medullary bone increases intra-osseous pressure and can promote an AVN focus.

Raised hydrostatic intra-medullary pressures have been further documented in relation with chronic alcoholism and corticosteroid therapy.

Perfusion of bone, as in every other organ depends on the difference between internal, i.e. intra-osseous, or arteriolar, and arterial pressures.

Treatment aimed at relieving this factor could be efficient only before extensive necrosis has taken place, i.e. in the up-slope of rising intra-medullary pressure and would be less effective in its plateau part and useless in its down-slope.

Vertebroplasty

Some therapies proposed by specialists are even contrary in their physiological concept to improvement of perfusion.

Such one is so-called *vertebroplasty*.

This technique consists in injecting through large bore needles glue into cancellous bone of vertebral bodies.

Advocated aim is filling vascular spaces therein with so much of this material as possible.

After my introduction in AVN, you would easily grasp the meaning, that such an event not only would not improve perfusion, but would worsen any setting of initial *Kümmel's disease*.

Thus, we (radiologists) see after such interventions *vertebra plana* cases more pronounced than ever witnessed previously or expected spontaneously.

Proponents' claims every pain subsides after this intervention is easily explained, as no nervous endings whatsoever survive complete necrosis inside vertebral bodies.

Anyway, to some point, AVN-focus has a natural tendency to extend, induced inflammatory reaction increasing hydrostatic pressure within bone.

Any situation of arterial hypotension, and especially those accompanied by centralization of vascular supply, as in shock syndromes, reduces medullary blood flow as well.

Architecture of bone

Local architecture of cancellous bone plays certainly a decisive role, as trabecular scaffold, which is meant to support body weight, is distributed unevenly, adapting itself to static and mechanic forces, after laws of physics.

Thicker and more numerous trabeculae leave less space for other components, especially in medullary bone, which are fat marrow, hematopoietic tissue and sinusoids: - This being the situation in cortical and sub-cortical areas (vertebral plateaus).

Thus not every part of a given osseous structure has the same chance to sustain a necrotic lesion.

Sub-cortical areas are probably dependent on their supply mainly on arterial support, while inside vertebrae, where sinusoids are numerous, and cancellous bone consists only of thin lamellae, bone is sustained by sinusoids themselves, and arterioles (on their venous side).

Thus, we can suspect, that there are two different ways of promoting AVN, one concerning sub-cortical bone is on arterial side of arterioles, the other one concerning central trabecular bone having its main issue on venous, which is sinusoidal side of arterioles.

Different mechanisms of AVN

Such a hypothesis is one attempt to explain different syndromes and clinical pictures of AVN.

It is well known that in the extremities ischemic lesions predominate in metaphyseal and epiphyseal parts, and especially in their sub-cortical counter-part, where trabecular bone contributes little to weight bearing.

In these locations thick cancellous lamellae take up torsion forces and distribute weight, leaving little space for sinusoids.

This is in contradistinction to diaphyseal portions, where supportive role is almost exclusively played by cortical bone and thus medullary infarcts are very rare.

Thus extremities have two counterparts for vertebral spine, one being sub-cortical areas, for instance in femoral head, known to harbor Perthes disease, the other one being transition between epiphysis and diaphysis, which is metaphysis, a complex bone architecture, not unlike vertebral medulla, frequent site of bone infarction as well, seen years after disease as central densification of spongiosa.

The situation seems to be more complex in

vertebral bodies, where subcortical areas are probably in an even higher risk situation for ischemia because of more tightly packed and thicker trabeculae.

This fact could be one explanation of biconcave, «fish vertebra» deformation.

In other words, there are probably at least two mechanisms which promote AVN:

- One responsible for subcortical lesions, as in Scheuermann's disease (Not unlike Legg-Calvé-Perthes disease), the other one locating centrally in bone, as in Kümmel's disease.

Thus, first one is illness of growing skeleton, due probably to rickets, while second one is pathology of the elderly person, due to osteoporosis.

Better adaptability of bone marrow in children in response to ischemic phenomena, than vertebral body fat in adults, could be one explanation for statistical discordance of those images.

As arterial blood flow is quite abundant in medullary space, the fact that a majority of ischemic lesions are observed in this location could mean that they have been induced rather by restriction on the venous or sinusoidal side.

Hypothesis for different physiopathology could imply facts like different remodeling mechanisms in cancellous (or spongious) and cortical bone.

Vertebral plates, being cortical bone, are thick lamellae, where giving on pressure could be interpreted as demand on nutriments and oxygen from arterial side, and where AVN appears only when supply is exceeded.

Center of vertebral bodies, being spongious bone, where cancellous lamellae are snugly coated by sinusoidal walls, are also remodeled by blood vessels, and especially venous channels.

In this location giving of scaffold to charges could be interpreted as chronically too high venous pressure, or high rate of remodeling of trabeculae.

Osteoporosis, which is main promoter of this image is end-result of chronic osteomalacia, on most occasions.

Two different components of bone

As bone lamellae resist to tension by their collagen matrix and to pressure by their mineral content, different qualitative defects of bone concerning those two main components would end-up probably in different patterns of bone remodeling on a microscopic level.

Imaging though doesn't show different behavior of vertebral bodies having in mind this dual nature of the weight supporting skeleton.

Scurvy, Marfan's disease, homocystinuria, Ehlers-Danlos disease and to a certain point osteogenesis imperfecta seem all to adopt the same imaging features in the vertebral spine as osteoporosis and osteomalacia or rickets do.

Thus production defects of the collagenous matrix or mineral content insufficiency end-up, because of other reasons, pertaining to bone synthesis, in a similar common pathway, being almost indistinguishable from each other by gross macroscopic features in the vertebral body picture.

This fact is easily explained by preceding considerations, on types of lamellar bone, thickness impediment whether due to defect in collagen matrix or mineral material having similar end-result.

Two different patterns in peripheral skeleton

This happens in contradistinction to the peripheral skeleton where stress which ends in insufficiency fractures involves mostly the concave curvature of long bones in true osteoporosis, rickets and osteomalacia and the convex counterpart of diaphysis in synthesis defects of collagen.

Precise radiological diagnosis of these diseases relies thus mainly on associated symptoms and signs in most cases, which are difficult to obtain by imaging of the vertebral spine alone.

As there is a minor trauma frequently associated with an evolving osteonecrosis in the spine, we can assume that oxygen demand in this context outgrows already limited supply reserves.

Observation with MRI suggests that minor trauma frequently induces a «bone bruise», which corresponds to micro-fractures in cancellous bone.

Eventually a tentative reparative process which ensues, provokes explosion of nutritive requirement.

As supply can't follow increasing demand, bone necrosis is promoted, resulting in vertebral body collapse.[1]

Ischemic survival of bone components

On microscopic level damage mechanisms in bone are relatively predictable:[2, 16]

- After an initial ischemic insult, myeloid cell death ensues within 6 to 12 hours.
- Osteocytes die in 48 hours.
- Lipocytes survive for up to 2-6 days.

Hyperemic bone response follows as a tentative reparative process, hyper-vascularity being limited by underlying disease.

Resorption of necrotic bone can occur only after repopulation with phagocytes, osteocytes, osteoclasts and osteoblasts has taken place.

It is these cells which restore viable bone.

Granulation tissue at first, and then new bone replace necrotic parts.

When a singular event of AVN takes place, it distributes in a pattern where a central focus of complete necrosis is surrounded by different lower degrees of damage.

Repopulation and the resulting reparative process would proceed in this model from the periphery towards the center.

- Imaging thus shows several areas in concentric arrangement around an AVN focus, and which relate to different levels and proportions of ischemia and resulting reparative process. (Fig 12)

Imaging of AVN

The most central part represents pure necrosis not reached by blood supply yet and thus without enhancement after intravenous contrast application.

Around this focus are disposed zones of progressive repopulation and incomplete cell death, and a «front line» of revascularization distinct by its intense enhancement, as well as different arrangement of bone trabeculae, new bone following a less force-oriented pattern of cancellous scaffold.

Of course more complex patterns can present owing to repetitive and multifocal AVN.

Different infarction types

Vascular blockade can take place on the arterial or venous side of intraosseous blood circulation.

While impeding venous return would promote a «red infarction» containing blood end products, arterial compromise would favor a «white infarction».

This reasonably implies two diametric different images.

Surprisingly, to my knowledge, this aspect hasn't been addressed as yet with modern imaging modalities in any publication so far.

Thus, if we try to understand this topic, we can imagine, that arterial compromise would shorten life of collagen matrix, and promote bending of vertebral plateaus; (Cortical bone).

This picture is more frequently observed when nutritional demand exceeds arterial blood support and flow. (Fast growing skeleton, f.i.)

While traumatic event of spine can impede with central venous flow through thrombosis;

And then resorption of this compound, after a few days, would take away essential trabeculae from spongy centrum, - End-result being flattening of vertebral body. (Cancellous bone).

Conclusion

In **conclusion** I can say that rather than a disease entity, AVN should be understood as an end result of many different pathological processes.

It is probably much more frequent than generally assumed, and represents a common pathway of bone reaction to many different diseases and conditions.

Only modern imaging, and especially MR allows disclosure of typical early changes (Fig 12).

In clinical practice, depicting findings which evoke the possibility of AVN should prompt further investigation in search for underlying disease and etiology.

Sometimes therapy should be warranted in order to prevent height loss, vertebral body deformation, and static instability of the vertebral spine and aimed also at relieving bothersome symptomatology.

Despite multiple causes, AVN of vertebral bodies assumes several typical patterns, which should be recognized and interpreted correctly.

Every radiologist should be aware of those characteristic images.

Any atypical features could mean a complication,

as for instance superinfection, especially in the clinical setting of sickle cell disease, and would need appropriate emergency therapy, adapted individually to every single situation.

References:

1. Antonucci MD et al, A histologic study of fractured human vertebral bodies in J Spinal Disord Tech 2002 Apr 15 (2): 118- 26
2. Assonline-Dayan Y et al, Pathogenesis and natural history of osteonecrosis. Semin Arthritis Rheum 2002 Oct; 32(2): 94-124
3. Begue P et al, Severe infections in children with sickle cell disease: clinical aspects and prevention. Arch Pediatr 2001 Sep 8 Suppl 4: 732s- 741s
4. Caffey's Pediatric X- Ray Diagnosis, 8th edition 1985, by Frederic N. Silverman, Year Book Medical Publ Inc.
5. Calza L et al, Osteonecrosis in HIV-infected patients and its correlation with highly active antiretroviral therapy (HAART), Presse Med 2003 Apr 5; 32(13Pt 1): 595-8

6.   Dupuy DE et al, Vertebral fluid collection associated with vertebral collapse. AJR 1996 Dec; 167(6): 1535-8

7.   Kümmel H, Die rarefizierende Ostitis der Wirbelkörper. Dtsch Med 1895, 21: 180-81

8.   Maldague BE et al, The intravertebral vacuum cleft: a sign of ischemic vertebral collapse. Radiology 1978; 129: 23-29

9.   Malghem J et al, Intravertebral vacuum cleft: changes in content after supine positioning. Radiology 1993 May, 187 (2): 483-7

10.   Murray RO, The radiology of skeletal disorders. 3rd edition 1991 Churchill Livingstone

11.   Naul LG, Avascular necrosis of the vertebral body: MR imaging; Radiology 1989 Jul; 172 (1): 219-22

12.   Olatunji AA et al, Sludge, stones and sickle cell anemia. Niger Postgrad Med J 2002 Dec; 9(4): 186-8

13.   Panow C et al, A case of aseptic vertebral necrosis in the context of metastatic lumbar disease. Neuroradiology

14.   Phemister DB, Necrotic bone and the subsequent changes which it undergoes, JAMA 1915; 64: 211

15.   Resnick D, Niwayama G, Intravertebral disc herniations: cartilaginous (Schmorl's) nodes. Radiology 1978, 126: 57-65

16. Resnick D, Diagnosis of bone and joint disorders. 3rd edition 1995 W. B. Saunders comp.

17. Scheuermann H, Kyphosis dorsalis juvenalis. Ugerskr Laeger 1920, 82: 384-93

18. Schmorl G, Junghans H, The human spine in health and disease, 2nd edn 1971, Grune&Stratton, New York, pp 3-41

19. Sedat-Ali M et al, The spine in sickle cell disease. Int Orthop 1994 Jun; 18(3): 154-6

20. Tauchmanova L et al, Avascular necrosis in long-term survivors after allogeneic or autologous stem cell transplantation: a single center experience and review, Cancer 2003 May 15; 97(10): 2453-61

21. Tectonidon MG et al, Asymptomatic vascular necrosis in patients with primary antiphospholipid syndrome in the absence of corticosteroid use: a prospective study by MRI. Arthritis Rheum 2003 Mar, 48(3): 732-6

22. Vogler JB 3rd et al, Bone marrow imaging, Radiology 1988; 168: 679-93

23. Weissman DE et al, Bone marrow necrosis in lymphoma studied by magnetic resonance imaging. Am J Hematol 1992 May; 40 (1): 42-6

24. Wright J et al, Septicemia caused by salmonella infection: an overlooked

complication of sickle cell disease. J Pediatr
1997 Mar; 130(3): 350-1

Figures, Drawings:

1.) «Fish vertebra» configuration. This pattern is typical of osteoporosis, but can also be found in other entities, especially diseases accompanied by bone marrow infiltration with pathological cells, as Gaucher's disease, multiple myeloma, sickle cell disease and other hemopathies.

2.) Schmorl's node: any off-center impression of the vertebral plateaus. This aspect has been described as a sign of Scheuermann's disease, but is not specific and can be found in other entities, for instance osteoporosis.

3.) Unequal size of adjacent vertebrae. Usually the vertebral size is even. That means that the size of every single vertebral body in any direction lies between the sizes of the two adjacent neighbor vertebrae.

4.) Similar to 3.) In this drawing the central vertebral body has outgrown its two neighbor vertebrae in transverse diameter. This feature is typical of Scheuermann's disease, but can also be observed on some bone dysplasias.

5.) Irregularities of the vertebral plateaus, which has been reported in Scheuermann's disease, but can also be seen in some dysplasias of bone and rarely in osteoporosis.

6.) Cuneiform deformation is also a typical feature of Scheuermann's disease but is specific only if combined with other signs. Isolated from clinical history and radiological context vertebral body cuneiform deformation represents a completely non-specific finding, as even compression fractures have the same appearance.

7.) Kümmel's disease is indistinguishable from compression fracture and often misdiagnosed as such. Vertebral body deformation appears however in Kümmel's disease delayed, several days after inducing traumatic event.

8.) Vertebra plana: represents one end of the spectrum of traumatic and infiltrative processes. This appearance is probably in most cases the end result of extensive bone necrosis.

9.) Vacuum cleft in a crushed vertebral body is one of the first specific signs of bone necrosis that has been reported in world literature.

10.) Photopenic center of concerned vertebral bodies observed in nuclear medicine. This finding in the acute stage of AVN can be very faint, depending on imaging modality, and can be easily overlooked.

11.)   Central T2-hyperintensity in necrotic collapsed vertebral body has been first described as a specific sign of AVN with MR-imaging.

12.)   This drawing represents T2-weighted, sagittal plane of vertebral spine. Central T1- and T2-hypointensity and absent enhancement of the same zone, are observed in necrosis of vertebral body as early signs, preceding deformation. This is probably an example of a «red infarction» of the vertebral body, owing to compromise in venous flow.

Fig. 1.

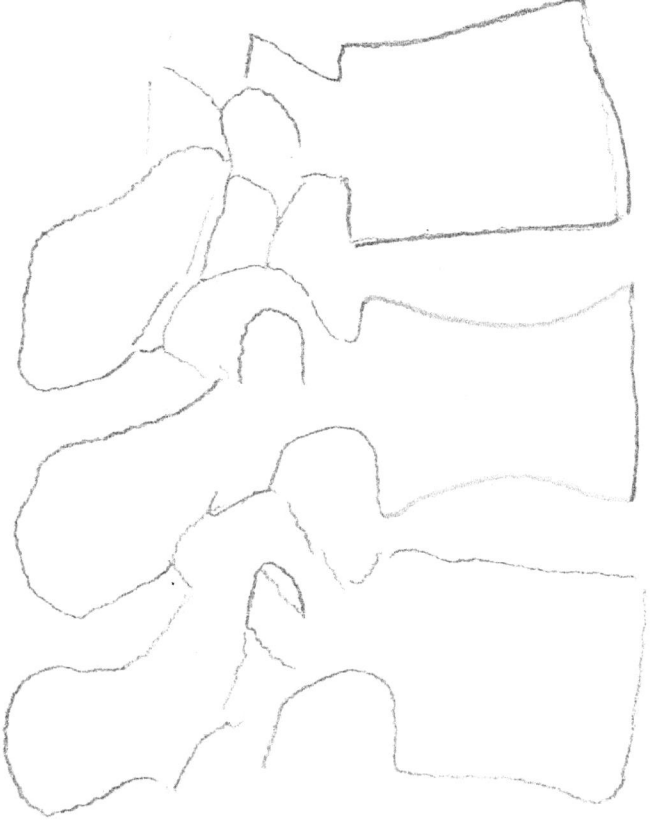

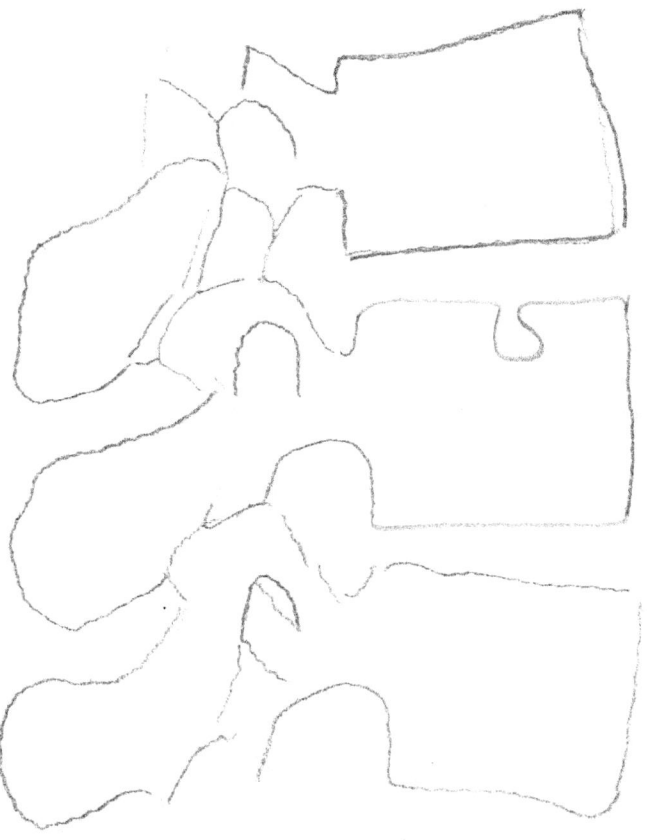

Fig. 2.

Fig. 3.

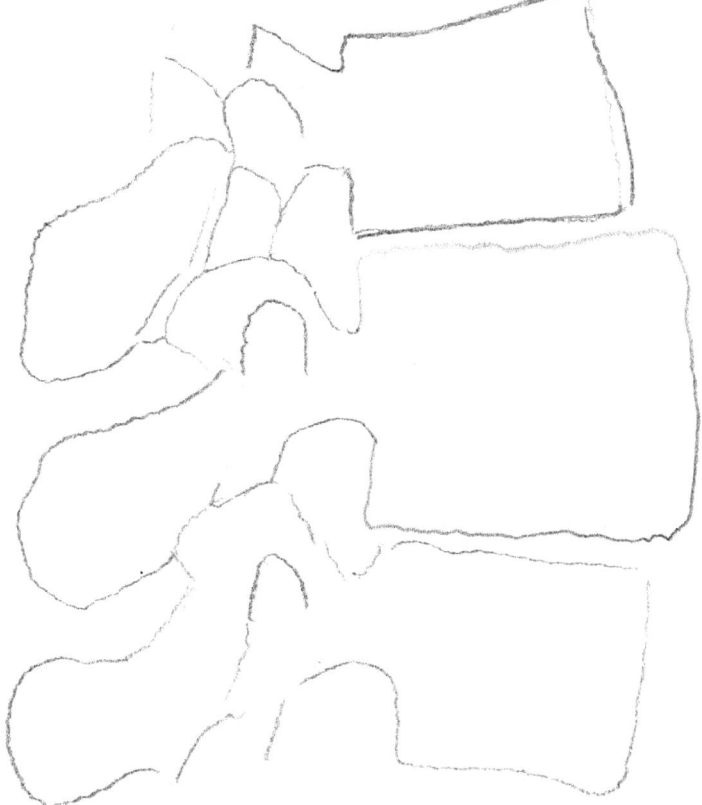

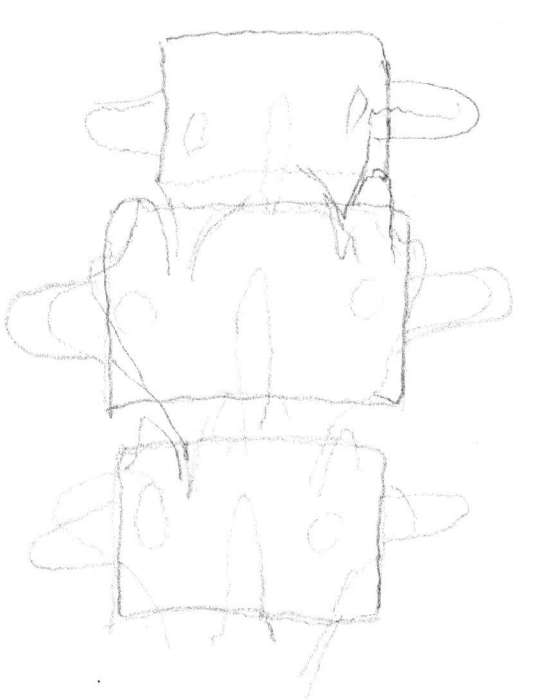

Fig. 4.

Fig. 5.

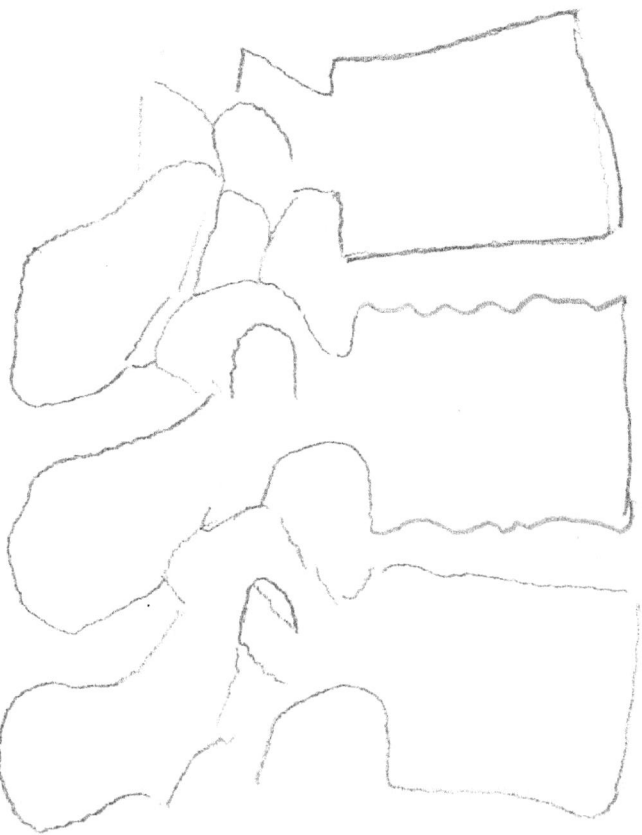

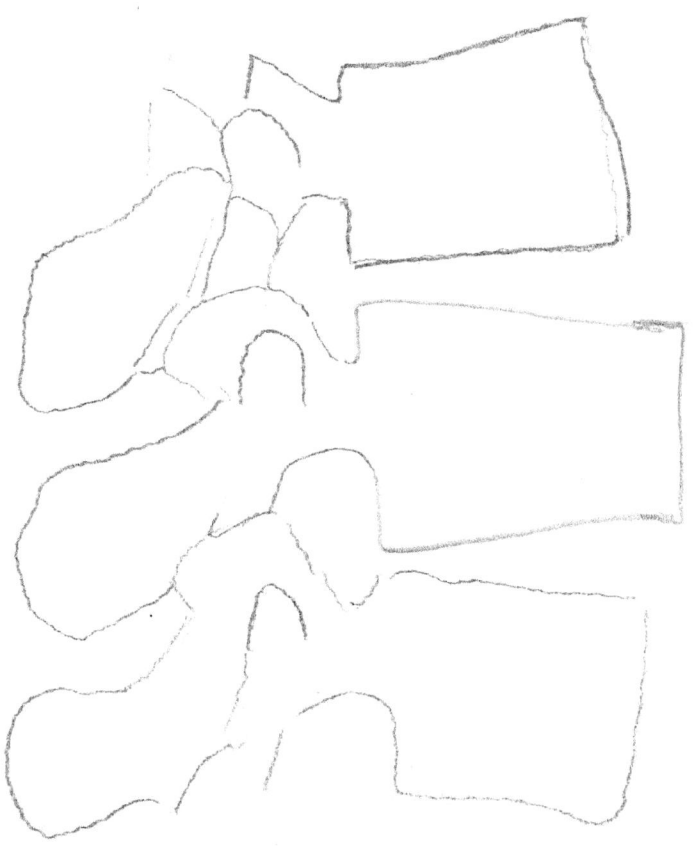

Fig. 6.

Fig. 7.

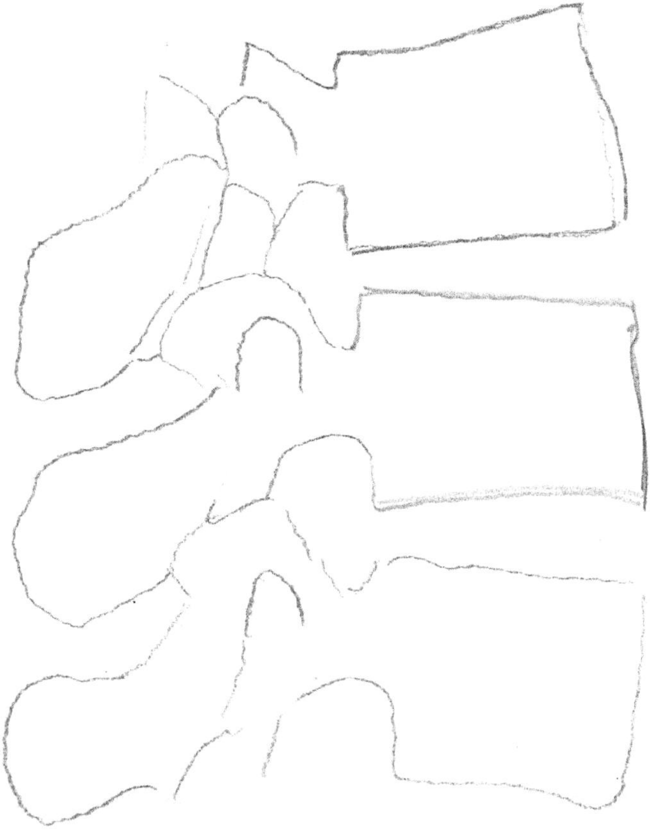

Fig. 8

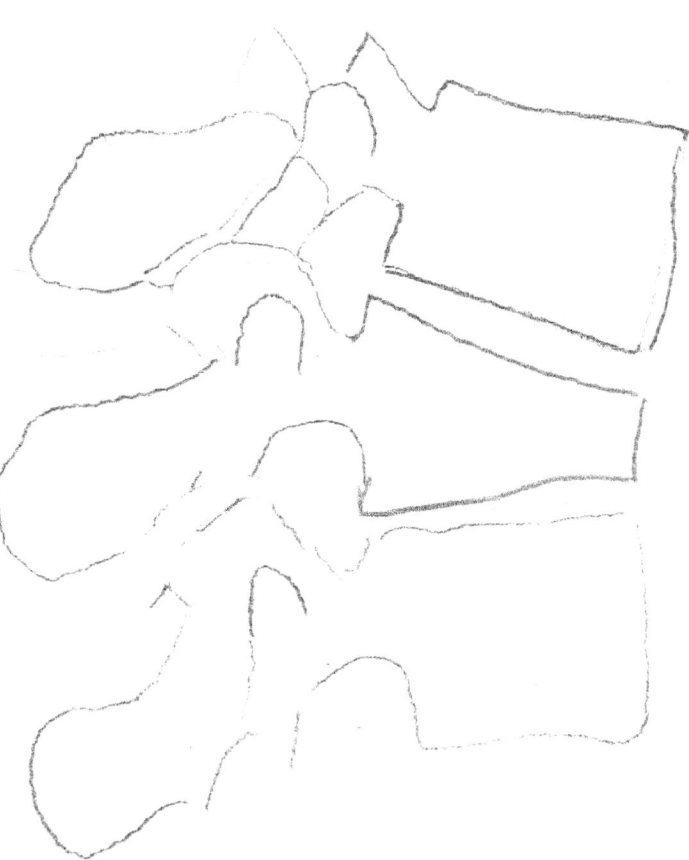

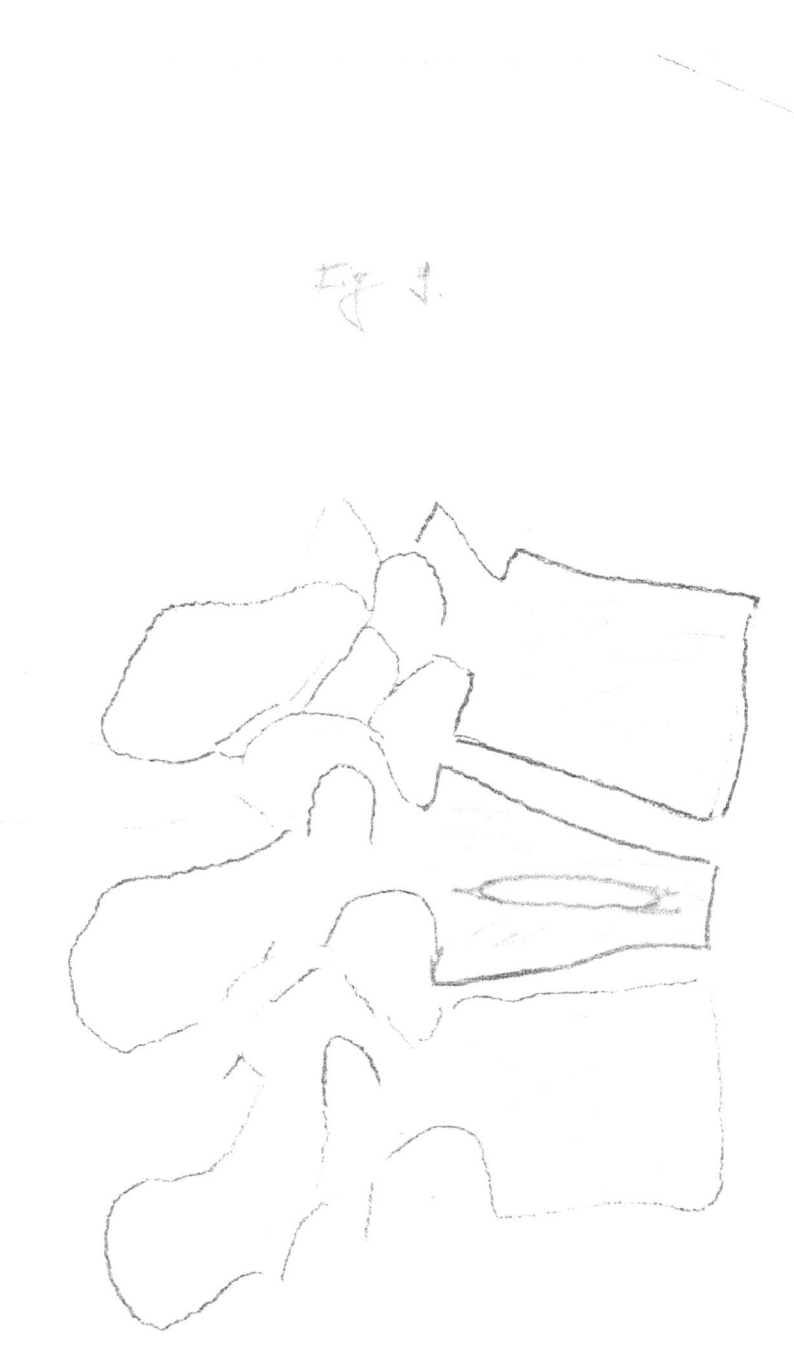

Fig 4.

Fig. 10.

Fig. 11.

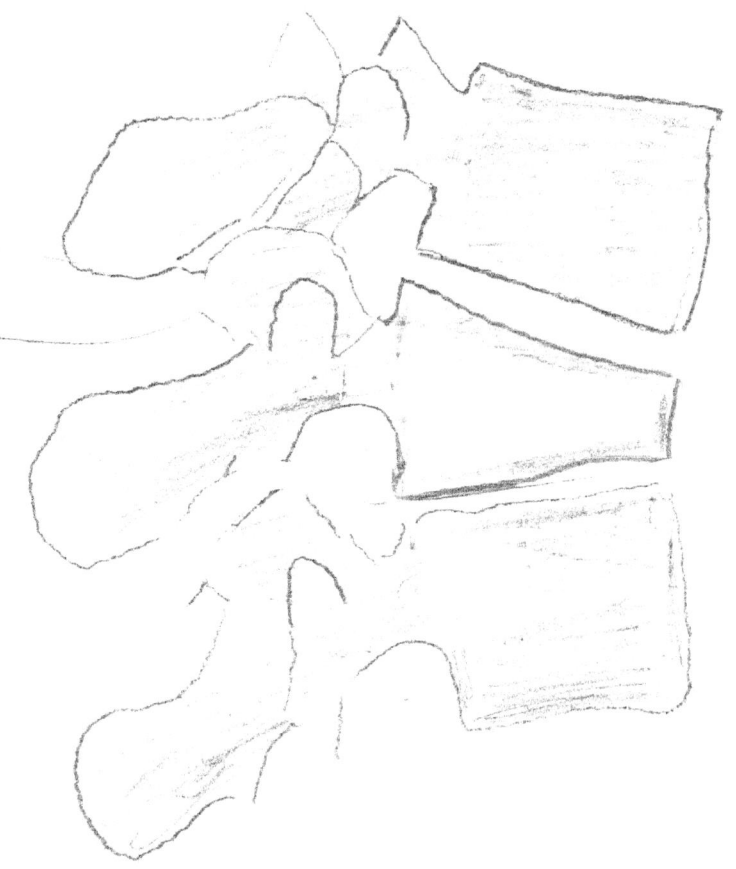

Fig 12.

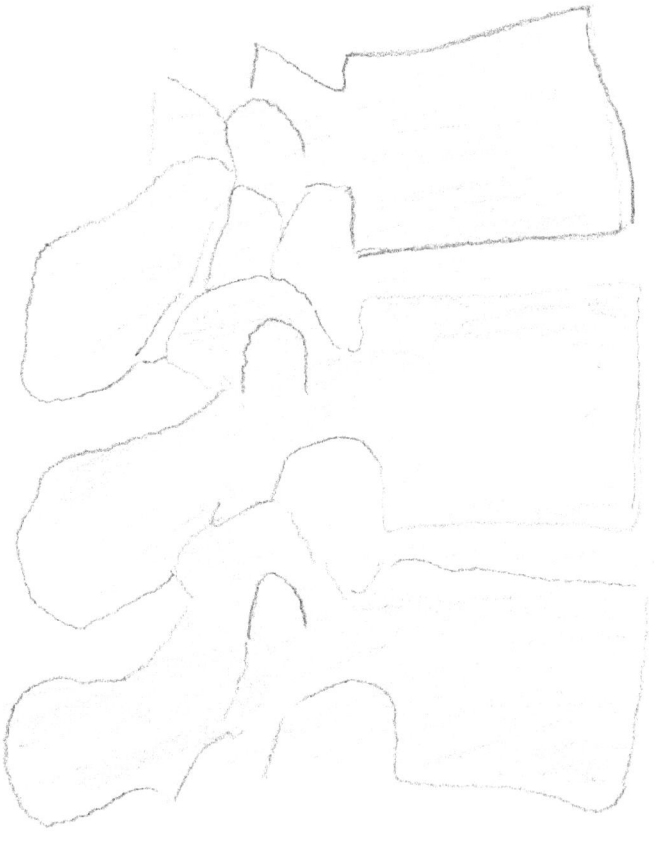